Unlocking Vibrant Health

The Rainbow Diet Journey to a Colorful and Nourished Life!"

Stephanie C. Levine

Copyright

Table of Contents

Conclusion

Acknowledgments

Introduction

Ever wondered if the secret to optimal health lies not in a pill or a fad diet but in the vibrant colors that grace your plate? Welcome to "Unlocking Vibrant Health:The Rainbow Diet Journey to a Colorful and Nourished Life!"Through the prism of the Rainbow Diet method, we set out on a transforming journey towards optimal health and well-being in this book.

At the heart of our journey lies the Rainbow Diet philosophy, a vibrant and holistic approach to nutrition that celebrates the diversity of colorful fruits and vegetables. Each hue represents a unique set of phytonutrients, antioxidants, vitamins, and minerals essential for nourishing our bodies and promoting vitality.

The rich crimson of tomatoes, strawberries, and red peppers signifies the presence of lycopene, a powerful antioxidant known for its potential to reduce the risk of chronic diseases such as heart disease and certain cancers. Incorporating red foods into our diet can enhance cardiovascular health and support overall well-being. Vibrant oranges, golden mangoes, and sunny bell peppers are bursting with beta-carotene, a precursor to vitamin A crucial for maintaining healthy vision, immune function, and skin integrity. By incorporating orange and yellow foods into our meals, we nourish our bodies with essential nutrients that promote immune resilience and glowing health. Verdant leafy greens like spinach, kale, and broccoli offer an abundance of chlorophyll, vitamins, and minerals that support detoxification, digestion, and cellular rejuvenation. The chlorophyll in green foods acts as a potent cleanser, helping to purify the bloodstream and enhance energy levels, while also providing an array of nutrients vital for optimal health.

Indigo-blueberries, royal purple grapes, and deep-hued eggplants are packed with anthocyanins, flavonoids that possess potent antioxidant and anti-inflammatory properties. Consuming blue and purple foods can help protect against oxidative stress, promote brain health, and reduce the risk of age-related cognitive decline, fostering vitality and cognitive function.white and brown foods such as garlic, onions, mushrooms, and whole grains offer a treasure trove of nutrients, including allicin, selenium, and fiber, essential for immune support, gut health, and balanced blood sugar levels. Incorporating these foods into our diet can bolster our body's defenses and provide sustained energy for optimal functioning.

By embracing the Rainbow Diet approach to nutrition, we embark on a journey of culinary exploration and nourishment, savoring the abundance of nature's palette while reaping the myriad health benefits each hue has to offer. Join us as we unlock the secrets to vibrant health and vitality, one colorful meal at a time. Remember, a rainbow Diet isn't a quick fix but a long-term lifestyle. Are you ready to embark on your Rainbow Diet journey? Let's dive in and unlock the vibrant health that awaits!

Chapter 1
Red Radiance - Exploring the Power of Antioxidant-Rich Red Foods

In this chapter, we delve into the significance of incorporating antioxidant-rich red foods into our diet. Red foods not only add color to our plates but also offer a plethora of health benefits that contribute to our overall well-being.

1. Understanding Antioxidants:

Before we dive into the specifics of red foods, it's essential to grasp the concept of antioxidants. Antioxidants are substances that assist in scavenging dangerous free radicals from our systems. Free radicals are unstable molecules that can cause oxidative stress, leading to cellular damage and various health issues. By consuming foods rich in antioxidants, such as those found in red fruits and vegetables, we can combat oxidative stress and promote optimal health.

2. The Power of Red:

Red foods derive their vibrant hue from phytonutrients such as lycopene, anthocyanins, and flavonoids, which possess potent antioxidant properties. These compounds not only give red foods their characteristic color but also contribute to their health-promoting abilities.

3. Exploring Red Foods:

A. Tomatoes:

Tomatoes are a rich source of lycopene, a powerful antioxidant known for its role in reducing the risk of chronic diseases such as heart disease and certain types of cancer.

Incorporating tomatoes into your diet, whether fresh, cooked, or in the form of sauces and soups, can provide numerous health benefits.

Nutritional Benefits:

✓ **Rich in Vitamin C:**

Tomatoes are an excellent source of vitamin C, which supports immune function and skin health.

✓ **High in Potassium:**

They contain potassium, which helps regulate blood pressure and muscle function.

✓ **Good Source of Folate:**

Folate, found in tomatoes, is important for DNA synthesis and cell division, making it especially beneficial during pregnancy.

✓ Provides Vitamin K:

Tomatoes contain vitamin K, which is essential for blood clotting and bone health.

✓ Low in Calories:

With only around 22 calories per 100 grams, tomatoes are a low-calorie option for those watching their weight.

✓ High in Water Content:

Their high water content helps keep you hydrated and contributes to feelings of fullness.

✓ Promotes Eye Health:

They are a good source of beta-carotene and lutein, which are beneficial for eye health and may reduce the risk of age-related macular degeneration.

✓ Supports Digestive Health:
Tomatoes contain fiber, which aids in digestion and promotes regular bowel movements.

✓ May Reduce Inflammation:
Tomatoes may help reduce inflammation in the body, potentially lowering the risk of chronic diseases like arthritis.

B. Red Bell Peppers:
Red bell peppers are packed with vitamin C, another antioxidant that supports immune function, skin health, and collagen production.

Additionally, they contain carotenoids like beta-carotene, which promote eye health and protect against age-related macular degeneration.

Nutritional Benefits:

✓ **High in Vitamin C:**
Red bell peppers are an excellent source of vitamin C, which is essential for immune function, skin health, and wound healing.

✓ **Rich in Antioxidants:**
They contain powerful antioxidants like carotenoids and flavonoids, which help protect cells from damage caused by free radicals.

✓ **Good Source of Vitamin A:**

Red bell peppers are rich in beta-carotene, which the body converts into vitamin A. The immune system, skin, and vision all benefit from vitamin A.

✓ **Low in Calories:**

They are low in calories, making them a great option for those looking to manage their weight.

✓ **High in Fiber:**

Red bell peppers are a good source of dietary fiber, which is important for digestive health and may help reduce the risk of certain chronic diseases.

✓ **Contains Vitamin B6:**

They provide a significant amount of vitamin B6, which is involved in energy metabolism and brain health.

✓ **Rich in Potassium:**

Red bell peppers are a good source of potassium, an essential mineral that helps regulate blood pressure and fluid balance in the body.

✓ **Promotes Eye Health:**

The high levels of vitamin A and other antioxidants in red bell peppers support eye health and may help reduce the risk of age-related macular degeneration.

✓ **Anti-Inflammatory Properties:**

Some compounds in red bell peppers have been found to have anti-inflammatory effects, which may help reduce the risk of chronic diseases like heart disease and arthritis.

✓ **May Aid in Cancer Prevention:**

The antioxidants and phytochemicals in red bell peppers may help protect against certain types of cancer by neutralizing free radicals and reducing inflammation.

C. Berries:

Varieties such as strawberries, raspberries, and cherries are not only delicious but also rich in anthocyanins, flavonoids, and vitamin C. These compounds help reduce inflammation, support cardiovascular health, and enhance cognitive function.

Nutritional Benefits:

✓ **Rich in Antioxidants:**

Berries contain high levels of antioxidants, such as anthocyanins, which help protect cells from damage caused by free radicals.

✓ **Vitamins and Minerals:**

Berries are packed with essential vitamins and minerals like vitamin C, vitamin K, manganese, and folate, which are important for overall health and immunity.

✓ **Fiber:**

They are a good source of dietary fiber, which aids in digestion, promotes gut health, and helps regulate blood sugar levels.

✓ **Heart Health:**

The flavonoids found in berries have been linked to improved heart health by reducing risk factors like high blood pressure and inflammation.

✓ **Weight Management:**

Berries are low in calories and high in fiber, making them a satisfying snack that can help with weight management and control.

✓ **Lower Risk of Chronic Diseases:**

Regular consumption of berries has been associated with a reduced risk of chronic diseases such as type 2 diabetes, certain cancers, and cardiovascular diseases.

✓ **Skin Health:**

The antioxidants in berries can help combat oxidative stress and promote skin health by reducing signs of aging and improving skin elasticity.

✓ Anti-Inflammatory Properties:

Berries contain compounds that have anti-inflammatory properties, which can help reduce inflammation in the body and alleviate symptoms of inflammatory conditions.

✓ Eye Health:

The antioxidants lutein and zeaxanthin found in berries may contribute to eye health by protecting against age-related macular degeneration and cataracts.

D. Beets:

Beets are renowned for their deep red color, which comes from betalains, a unique class of antioxidants. Betalains possess anti-inflammatory and detoxifying properties, making beets a valuable addition to any diet.

Nutritional Benefits:

✓ Rich in Nutrients:

Beets are packed with essential vitamins and minerals such as folate, manganese, potassium, and vitamin C.

✓ High in Fiber:

Beets are a good source of dietary fiber, which can aid digestion and promote a healthy gut.

✓ Heart Health:

The nitrates in beets can help lower blood pressure and improve overall heart health.

✓ **Antioxidant Properties:**

Beets contain antioxidants like betalains, which help protect cells from damage caused by free radicals.

✓ **Anti-Inflammatory:**

Betaine, a compound found in beets, has been shown to have anti-inflammatory properties, potentially reducing the risk of chronic diseases.

✓ **Supports Liver Health:**

Betaine also supports liver function by helping to reduce fatty deposits in the liver and promoting detoxification.

✓ **Boosts Exercise Performance:**

The nitrates in beets may improve exercise performance by enhancing oxygen utilization and increasing endurance.

✓ **May Help Lower Blood Sugar:**

Beetroot juice may help regulate blood sugar levels, though more research is needed.

✓ **Promotes Weight Loss:**

Beets are low in calories and high in water content, making them a filling and nutritious option for those trying to lose weight.

✓ **Brain Health:**

The nitrates in beets may improve blood flow to the brain, potentially enhancing cognitive function and reducing the risk of age-related cognitive decline.

E. Red Apples:

Apples contain quercetin, a flavonoid with antioxidant and anti-inflammatory effects. Consuming red apples can help lower cholesterol levels, regulate blood sugar, and promote gut health.

Nutritional Benefits:

✓ Rich in Fiber:

Red apples are a good source of dietary fiber, which aids in digestion and helps maintain bowel regularity.

✓ Low in Calories:

They are low in calories, making them a great snack option for those looking to manage their weight.

✓ Packed with Vitamins:

Red apples contain essential vitamins such as Vitamin C, which supports the immune system, and Vitamin A, which is beneficial for eye health.

✓ Antioxidant Properties:

These apples are rich in antioxidants like quercetin, which helps protect cells from damage caused by free radicals.

✓ Heart Health:

The soluble fiber in red apples can help lower cholesterol levels, reducing the risk of heart disease.

✓ **Blood Sugar Regulation:**

The fiber and natural sugars in red apples can help regulate blood sugar levels, making them a suitable choice for diabetics when consumed in moderation.

✓ **Hydration:**

Red apples have high water content, helping to keep you hydrated.

✓ **Bone Health:**

They contain trace amounts of minerals like calcium and potassium, which are essential for bone health.

✓ Improved Gut Health:

The combination of fiber and natural sugars in red apples can promote the growth of beneficial gut bacteria, supporting overall gut health.

✓ Cancer Prevention:

Antioxidants and phytochemicals found in red apples may have protective effects against certain types of cancer.

4. Incorporating Yellow Foods into Your Diet:

Now that we understand the nutritional benefits of red foods, it's time to incorporate them into our daily meals. Try adding a variety of red fruits and vegetables to salads, smoothies, and stir-fries, or simply enjoy them as snacks.

Experiment with different recipes to discover delicious ways to harness the power of red for vibrant health. By incorporating tomatoes, red bell peppers, berries, beets, and red apples into our diet, we can harness the power of phytonutrients to combat oxidative stress, reduce inflammation, and support overall well-being. Stay tuned for the next chapter, where we'll delve into the benefits of orange foods on our Rainbow Diet journey!

Chapter 2
Orange Glow - Harnessing the Energy and Vitality of Orange-Colored Nutrients

In this chapter, we embark on the exploration of orange-colored nutrients and their profound impact on our well-being. From the vibrant hue of oranges to the earthy glow of sweet potatoes, the spectrum of orange foods offers a treasure trove of nutrients essential for optimal health.

1. The Significance of Orange-Colored Nutrients:

Orange-colored fruits and vegetables are rich in carotenoids, particularly beta-carotene, which the body converts into vitamin A. This vital nutrient plays a crucial role in maintaining healthy vision, supporting immune function, and promoting skin health. Additionally, orange foods are abundant in antioxidants, such as vitamin C, which help combat oxidative stress and inflammation, reducing the risk of chronic diseases like heart disease and cancer.

2. Exploring Orange-Colored Foods:

A. Oranges:

Bursting with vitamin C and fiber, oranges are not only refreshing but also promote heart health and aid in digestion. Incorporating oranges into your diet can help lower cholesterol levels and support healthy blood pressure.

Nutritional Benefits:

✓ **Vitamin C:**

Oranges are rich in vitamin C, which supports the immune system, promotes wound healing, and helps the body absorb iron.

✓ **Fiber:**

Oranges contain dietary fiber, which aids digestion, helps prevent constipation, and supports overall gut health.

✓ **Antioxidants**:

Oranges are packed with antioxidants like flavonoids, carotenoids, and vitamin C, which help protect cells from damage caused by free radicals.

✓ **Hydration:**

Oranges are high in water content, helping to keep you hydrated and maintain fluid balance in the body.

✓ Potassium:

Oranges are a good source of potassium, an essential mineral that helps regulate blood pressure, muscle contractions, and nerve function.

✓ Folate:

Oranges contain folate, a B-vitamin important for cell division and DNA synthesis, making it crucial during pregnancy for proper fetal development.

✓ Vitamin A:

Oranges provide vitamin A in the form of beta-carotene, which is important for vision health, immune function, and skin health.

✓ **Calcium**:

Oranges contain calcium, which is essential for bone health, muscle function, and nerve transmission.

✓ **Thiamine (Vitamin B1):**

Oranges contain thiamine, a B vitamin that helps convert food into energy and supports nerve function.

✓ **Magnesium**:

Oranges provide magnesium, an essential mineral involved in over 300 biochemical reactions in the body, including energy production and muscle function.

B. Carrots:

Known for their high beta-carotene content, carrots are a powerhouse of nutrients. They promote eye health, boost immune function, and contribute to glowing skin. Moreover, their crunchy texture makes them a satisfying snack option.

Nutritional Benefits:

✓ **Rich in Vitamin A:**

Carrots are loaded with beta-carotene, a precursor of vitamin A, which is essential for maintaining good vision, especially in low-light conditions.

✓ **Antioxidant Properties:**

Carrots contain antioxidants like beta-carotene, alpha-carotene, and lutein, which help protect the body from oxidative stress and reduce the risk of chronic diseases.

✓ **Supports Eye Health:**

Beta-carotene in carrots is converted into vitamin A in the body, which is crucial for maintaining healthy eyesight and preventing conditions like night blindness and age-related macular degeneration.

✓ **Boosts Immunity:**

Carrots are rich in various vitamins and minerals, including vitamin C, which helps strengthen the immune system and protects the body against infections.

✓ Promotes Digestive Health:

The dietary fiber in carrots promotes regular bowel movements, prevents constipation, and supports a healthy digestive system.

✓ Heart Health:

Potassium and fiber in carrots help maintain healthy blood pressure levels and reduce the risk of heart disease by lowering cholesterol levels.

✓ May Reduce Cancer Risk:

Carrots contain antioxidants like beta-carotene and falcarinol, which may help reduce the risk of certain cancers, including lung, breast, and colon cancer.

✓ Aids in Weight Loss:

Carrots are low in calories and high in fiber, making them a great snack option for those trying to lose weight as they can help keep you full for longer periods.

✓ Promotes Skin Health:

The beta-carotene in carrots helps protect the skin from sun damage and promotes healthy skin by preventing premature aging and improving skin tone.

✓ Supports Oral Health:

Chewing on raw carrots stimulates the production of saliva, which helps maintain oral hygiene by reducing the risk of cavities and removing plaque from teeth.

C. Sweet Potatoes:

These nutrient-dense root vegetables are packed with beta-carotene, vitamin C, and fiber. Sweet potatoes provide sustained energy, support gut health, and contribute to healthy aging. Their versatility makes them a staple in various culinary creations.

Nutritional Benefits:

✓ **High in Fiber:**

Sweet potatoes are rich in dietary fiber, which aids in digestion and helps maintain bowel regularity.

✓ **Vitamins and Minerals:**

They are packed with essential vitamins and minerals, including vitamin A, vitamin C, potassium, and manganese, which support overall health and immune function.

✓ **Antioxidants**:

Sweet potatoes contain various antioxidants, such as beta-carotene, which can help reduce the risk of chronic diseases and protect cells from damage.

✓ **Low Glycemic Index:**

Despite their sweetness, sweet potatoes have a lower glycemic index compared to regular potatoes, meaning they have less of an impact on blood sugar levels.

✓ **Heart Health:**

The high levels of potassium in sweet potatoes can help regulate blood pressure and reduce the risk of heart disease.

✓ Anti-inflammatory Properties:

Certain compounds in sweet potatoes have anti-inflammatory properties, which may help reduce inflammation in the body and lower the risk of chronic diseases.

✓ Digestive Health:

The fiber content in sweet potatoes promotes a healthy digestive system by preventing constipation and supporting gut health.

✓ Weight Management:

Sweet potatoes are relatively low in calories and fat, making them a satisfying and nutritious option for those looking to manage their weight.

✓ Energy Production:

The complex carbohydrates in sweet potatoes provide a steady source of energy, making them an excellent choice for sustained energy throughout the day.

✓ Eye Health:

The beta-carotene in sweet potatoes is converted to vitamin A in the body, which is essential for maintaining healthy vision and may reduce the risk of age-related macular degeneration.

D. Mangoes:

With their luscious sweetness and vibrant color, mangoes are a tropical delight loaded with vitamin C, vitamin A, and antioxidants. Consuming mangoes promotes collagen formation, enhances immunity, and may even aid in weight management.

Nutritional Benefits:

✓ **Rich in Vitamins:**

Mangoes are packed with vitamins A, C, E, and K, which support various bodily functions including vision, immune health, and skin health.

✓ **High in Fiber:**

They are a good source of dietary fiber, aiding digestion, promoting gut health, and helping to prevent constipation.

✓ Antioxidant Properties:

Mangoes contain antioxidants like quercetin, astragalin, and beta-carotene, which help to neutralize free radicals in the body and protect against chronic diseases.

✓ Boosts Immunity:

The high vitamin C content in mangoes helps boost the immune system, aiding in the body's defense against infections and illnesses.

✓ Supports Heart Health:

Mangoes are rich in potassium, which helps regulate blood pressure and heart rate, reducing the risk of heart disease and stroke.

✓ **Improves Eye Health:**
The vitamin A content in mangoes promotes good vision and helps prevent age-related macular degeneration.

✓ **Enhances Skin Health:**
The vitamin E content in mangoes helps maintain healthy skin by protecting against UV radiation and promoting collagen production.

✓ **Aids Weight Loss:**
Despite being sweet, mangoes are relatively low in calories and fat, making them a good option for those looking to manage their weight.

✓ **Regulates Blood Sugar Levels:**

Mangoes have a low glycemic index, meaning they release sugar into the bloodstream slowly, helping to regulate blood sugar levels.

✓ **Promotes Bone Health:**

Mangoes contain vitamin K, which is important for bone health and helps in the absorption of calcium, essential for maintaining strong bones.

E. Papayas:

Rich in enzymes like papain, papayas support digestion and alleviate bloating. They are also a great source of vitamin C, vitamin A, and folate, offering numerous health benefits ranging from improved skin health to reduced inflammation.

Nutritional Benefits:

✓ **Rich in Vitamin C:**

Papayas are an excellent source of vitamin C, which helps boost the immune system and promotes healthy skin.

✓ **High in Fiber:**

They contain a good amount of dietary fiber, which aids digestion and promotes regular bowel movements.

✓ **Loaded with Antioxidants:**

Papayas are rich in antioxidants like carotenoids, flavonoids, and vitamin E, which help protect cells from damage caused by free radicals.

✓ **Contains Enzymes:**

Papayas contain enzymes like papain and chymopapain, which aid in digestion by breaking down proteins.

✓ Good for Eye Health:

They are a good source of beta-carotene, lutein, and zeaxanthin, which are beneficial for eye health and may reduce the risk of age-related macular degeneration.

✓ Support Heart Health:

Papayas are low in cholesterol and high in potassium, which helps regulate blood pressure and may reduce the risk of heart disease.

✓ Anti-inflammatory Properties:

The enzymes and antioxidants in papayas have anti-inflammatory properties, which may help reduce inflammation in the body.

✓ **Aids in Weight Loss:**

Due to their high fiber content and low-calorie count, papayas can be a satisfying and nutritious addition to a weight loss diet.

✓ **Supports Skin Health:**

Vitamin C and other antioxidants in papayas help promote collagen production, which keeps the skin firm and youthful.

3. Incorporating Yellow Foods into Your Diet:

To harness the energy and vitality of orange-colored nutrients, consider the following tips:

- Start your day with a refreshing glass of freshly squeezed orange juice or a colorful smoothie packed with mangoes and carrots.

- Incorporate roasted sweet potatoes into your salads, soups, or Buddha bowls for a hearty and nutritious meal.

- Snack on crunchy carrot sticks paired with hummus or enjoy slices of juicy papaya as a midday pick-me-up.

- Experiment with savory dishes featuring butternut squash or pumpkin, adding depth and flavor to your meals.

- Indulge in the natural sweetness of dried apricots or Medjool dates as a satisfying dessert alternative.

The radiant glow of orange-colored nutrients illuminates the path to vibrant health and vitality. By embracing the diverse array of fruits and vegetables within the orange spectrum, you can nourish your body, support your immune system, and enhance your overall well-being. Join us on this Rainbow Diet journey as we continue to unlock the secrets of optimal health one colorful nutrient at a time.

Chapter 3
Yellow Sunshine - Illuminating Health Benefits Through Yellow-Hued Foods

In this chapter, we will delve into the health benefits of yellow-hued foods, exploring how these vibrant ingredients can contribute to your overall well-being and vitality. Just like the warm rays of sunshine, yellow foods bring brightness and energy to your plate, nourishing your body from within. Let's embark on a journey to uncover the golden treasures of nutrition that lie within these radiant foods.

1. The Power of Yellow Foods:

Yellow foods are not only visually appealing but also packed with essential nutrients that promote optimal health. From vibrant fruits to hearty vegetables, the yellow spectrum offers a diverse array of flavors and textures, each contributing to your overall wellness in unique ways. Whether it's the vitamin C-rich citrus fruits or the beta-carotene-packed squash, incorporating yellow foods into your diet can have a profound impact on your vitality and longevity.

Examples of yellow fruits are: Banana, Lemon, Pineapple etc

2. Exploring yellow - Coloured food:

A. Bananas:

Nutritional Benefits:

✓ **Rich in Potassium:**

Bananas are high in potassium, which is essential for heart health, blood pressure regulation, and muscle function.

✓ **High in Fiber:**

They are a good source of dietary fiber, which aids digestion and promotes feelings of fullness

✓ **Vitamins and Minerals:**

Bananas contain vitamins C and B6, as well as various minerals like manganese and magnesium, which support overall health.

✓ **Energy Boost:**

They are a convenient and quick source of energy due to their natural sugars, especially glucose, fructose, and sucrose.

✓ **Heart Health:**

The potassium and fiber content in bananas may help lower the risk of heart disease by reducing blood pressure and improving cholesterol levels.

B. Pineapples:

Nutritional Benefits:

✓ **Rich in Vitamin C:**

Pineapples are packed with vitamin C, which boosts the immune system and aids in collagen production for healthy skin and joints.

✓ **Digestive Aid:**

They contain bromelain, an enzyme that aids digestion by breaking down proteins and reducing bloating.

✓ Anti-Inflammatory Properties:
Bromelain also has anti-inflammatory properties, potentially reducing pain and swelling associated with inflammatory conditions.

✓ Hydration:
Pineapples have high water content, helping to keep the body hydrated and maintain electrolyte balance

✓ Eye Health:
The high levels of antioxidants, such as beta-carotene, in pineapples may help prevent age-

related macular degeneration and promote overall eye health.

C. Lemon:

Nutritional Benefits:

✓ **High in Vitamin C:**
Lemons are a rich source of vitamin C, which is essential for immune function, skin health, and wound healing.

✓ **Antioxidant Properties:**
Lemons contain flavonoids, which are antioxidants that help protect cells from damage caused by free radicals.

✓ **Aids Digestion:**

The citric acid in lemons stimulates the production of digestive juices, which can help with digestion and prevent constipation.

✓ Alkalizing Effect:

Despite being acidic outside the body, lemons have an alkalizing effect when metabolized, which can help balance the body's pH levels.

✓ Potassium Content:

Lemons contain potassium, an essential mineral that helps regulate blood pressure and supports heart health.

3. Incorporating Yellow Foods into Your Diet:

Now that we've explored the numerous health benefits and nutritional benefits of yellow-hued foods, it's time to incorporate them into your daily meals.

Here are some simple and delicious ways to add a splash of sunshine to your diet:

- Start your day with a refreshing smoothie made with bananas and pineapples for a burst of vitamin C and potassium.

- Incorporate roasted sweet potatoes, carrots, and yellow bell peppers into hearty salads or nourishing grain bowls for a colorful and nutrient-rich meal.

- Experiment with turmeric in your cooking by adding it to soups, stews, or stir-fries for its vibrant color and anti-inflammatory properties.

- Snack on fresh slices of yellow watermelon or golden berries for a sweet and nutritious treat packed with antioxidants and vitamins.

Yellow foods offer a wealth of nutritional benefits that can enhance your overall health and well-being. From boosting immunity to supporting heart health and promoting digestive regularity, incorporating yellow-hued foods into your diet can help you unlock vibrant health and vitality. So, embrace the sunshine on your plate and savor the golden treasures of nutrition that these radiant foods have to offer on your Rainbow Diet journey to a colorful and nourished life!

Chapter 4
Green Vitality - Unveiling the Nutrient-Rich World of Green Superfoods

In this chapter, we delve into the vibrant world of green superfoods, exploring their immense nutritional value and the numerous health benefits they offer. From leafy greens to nutrient-packed vegetables, green superfoods are essential components of a balanced and nourishing diet. Let's embark on a journey to uncover the secrets of green vitality and learn how these powerful foods can transform your health and well-being.

1. The Power of Leafy Greens:

Nutritional Benefits:

✓ Rich in vitamins:

Leafy greens like spinach, kale, and Swiss chard are packed with vitamins A, C, and K, which are essential for maintaining overall health.

✓ High in fiber:

Leafy vegetables are an excellent source of dietary fiber, which aids digestion, promotes satiety, and supports a healthy gut microbiome.

✓ Low in calories:

Most leafy greens are low in calories, making them a great choice for weight management and calorie-conscious diets.

✓ Rich in antioxidants:

These vegetables are abundant in antioxidants like beta-carotene, lutein, and zeaxanthin, which help protect cells from damage caused by free radicals.

✓ **Good source of minerals:**

Leafy greens contain essential minerals such as iron, calcium, magnesium, and potassium, which are crucial for maintaining bone health, muscle function, and electrolyte balance.

✓ **Heart-healthy:**

The high levels of potassium and magnesium in leafy greens can help regulate blood pressure and support heart health.

✓ **Anti-inflammatory properties:**

Many leafy vegetables contain phytochemicals that possess anti-inflammatory properties, potentially reducing the risk of chronic diseases like heart disease and arthritis.

✓ Promote eye health:

Leafy greens are rich in lutein and zeaxanthin, antioxidants that are important for eye health and may help reduce the risk of age-related macular degeneration.

✓ Blood sugar regulation:

The fiber and antioxidants found in leafy greens can help stabilize blood sugar levels, making them beneficial for individuals with diabetes or those at risk of developing it.

✓ Boost immune function:

The vitamins and minerals present in leafy greens play a vital role in supporting a healthy immune system, helping the body fight off infections and illnesses.

Incorporating a variety of leafy greens into your diet can enhance immune function, promote healthy digestion, and support detoxification processes in the body.

2. Cruciferous Vegetables:

Nutritional Benefits:

✓ **Rich in Nutrients:**
Cruciferous vegetables like broccoli, cauliflower, and Brussels sprouts are packed

with essential vitamins and minerals, including vitamin C, vitamin K, folate, and potassium.

✓ High in Fiber:

They are excellent sources of dietary fiber, which promotes digestive health, helps regulate blood sugar levels, and supports weight management by promoting feelings of fullness.

✓ Antioxidant Properties:

Cruciferous vegetables contain antioxidants like beta-carotene and various flavonoids, which help protect cells from damage caused by free radicals and reduce the risk of chronic diseases.

✓ Cancer-Fighting Compounds:

Compounds like sulforaphane and indole-3-carbinol found in cruciferous vegetables have been linked to a reduced risk of certain cancers, including breast, prostate, and colon cancer.

✓ **Anti-inflammatory Effects:**

These vegetables contain compounds that have anti-inflammatory properties, which can help reduce inflammation in the body and lower the risk of chronic diseases associated with inflammation.

✓ **Heart Health Benefits:**

Regular consumption of cruciferous vegetables has been associated with a lower risk of heart disease due to their ability to reduce cholesterol levels, improve blood vessel function, and lower blood pressure.

✓ **Support Detoxification:**

Cruciferous vegetables contain sulfur-containing compounds that support the body's detoxification processes, aiding in the removal of harmful toxins and promoting overall health.

✓ **Weight Management**:

With their low calorie and high fiber content, cruciferous vegetables can be a valuable addition to a weight loss or weight management diet, helping to control appetite and reduce calorie intake.

✓ **Bone Health:**

Cruciferous vegetables are good sources of vitamin K, which plays a crucial role in bone health by supporting calcium absorption and reducing the risk of osteoporosis.

✓ **Gut Health:**

The fiber and phytonutrients in cruciferous vegetables promote a healthy gut microbiome, supporting digestive health and reducing the risk of gastrointestinal disorders like constipation and diverticulosis.

3. The Versatility of Green Herbs:

Nutritional Benefits:

Green herbs, such as parsley, cilantro, basil, mint, and others, offer numerous nutritional benefits:

✓ **Rich in Antioxidants:**

Green herbs are packed with antioxidants like flavonoids and polyphenols, which help combat

oxidative stress and reduce the risk of chronic
diseases.

✓ Vitamins and Minerals:

They are excellent sources of vitamins A, C, and
K, as well as minerals like calcium, iron,
magnesium, and potassium, crucial for various
bodily functions.

✓ Digestive Health:

Many green herbs contain compounds that aid
digestion, such as fiber and enzymes, promoting
gut health and reducing digestive discomfort.

✓ Anti-inflammatory Properties:

Certain green herbs possess anti-inflammatory
properties, which can help alleviate

inflammation in the body and reduce the risk of inflammatory conditions.

✓ Heart Health:

The high levels of antioxidants and potassium in green herbs may support heart health by lowering blood pressure, reducing cholesterol levels, and improving overall cardiovascular function.

✓ Immune System Support:

The vitamins and minerals found in green herbs play vital roles in supporting the immune system, helping the body defend against infections and illnesses.

✓ Detoxification:

Some green herbs, like cilantro, have been shown to aid in detoxifying the body by binding to heavy metals and assisting in their removal.

✓ Weight Management:

Green herbs are low in calories and rich in flavor, making them excellent additions to meals for adding taste without significantly increasing caloric intake, thus aiding in weight management.

✓ Bone Health:

The vitamin K content in green herbs contributes to bone health by assisting in calcium absorption and promoting bone density.

✓ Fresh Breath:

Many green herbs, such as parsley and mint, contain compounds that can help freshen breath and reduce the bacteria that cause bad breath. Incorporating fresh herbs into your meals not only enhances the taste but also boosts the nutritional value, making every dish a nourishing and flavorful experience.

4. Spirulina and Chlorella:

Nutritional Benefits:

✓ Protein-rich:

Both Spirulina and Chlorella are high in protein, making them excellent sources of plant-based protein, which is essential for muscle repair and growth.

✓ Vitamins:

They are rich in various vitamins, including vitamin A, vitamin C, vitamin E, and several B vitamins, which play crucial roles in maintaining overall health and supporting various bodily functions.

✓ Minerals:

Spirulina and Chlorella are abundant in minerals such as iron, calcium, magnesium, and potassium, which are essential for bone health, muscle function, and overall well-being.

✓ Antioxidants:

They contain potent antioxidants like beta-carotene, chlorophyll, and phycocyanin, which help combat oxidative stress and reduce inflammation in the body.

✓ **Omega-3 fatty acids**:

They provide a good source of omega-3 fatty acids, particularly alpha-linolenic acid (ALA), which supports heart health, and brain function, and reduces inflammation.

✓ **Detoxification:**

Both Spirulina and Chlorella have detoxifying properties, helping to remove heavy metals and toxins from the body, supporting liver health and overall detoxification processes.

✓ **Immune support:**

The rich array of nutrients in Spirulina and Chlorella, along with their antioxidant properties, can help strengthen the immune system and improve resistance to infections and illnesses.

✓ Energy boost:

Consuming Spirulina and Chlorella can increase energy levels and reduce fatigue due to their nutrient-dense composition, providing a natural boost to physical and mental vitality.

✓ Digestive health:

They contain fiber and chlorophyll, which support digestive health by promoting regularity, supporting healthy gut flora, and aiding in detoxification processes.

✓ Weight management:

Incorporating Spirulina and Chlorella into a balanced diet may aid in weight management due to their high protein content, ability to regulate blood sugar levels, and potential to increase feelings of satiety.

Adding spirulina and chlorella to your diet in the form of powder or tablets can provide a convenient and effective way to boost your nutrient intake and support optimal health.

Green superfoods are an essential component of a vibrant and nourished life. From leafy greens and cruciferous vegetables to green herbs and algae, these nutrient-rich foods offer a myriad of health benefits that support overall well-being. By incorporating a variety of green superfoods into your diet regularly, you can unlock the secret to vibrant health and vitality, paving the way to a colorful and nourished life

Chapter 5

Blue Indulgence - Diving into the Healthful Qualities of Blue and Purple Foods

Welcome to the vibrant world of blue and purple foods! In this chapter, we'll explore the rich array of nutrients and health benefits these colorful foods offer, and how they can contribute to your journey towards vibrant health.

Blue and purple foods encompass a diverse range of fruits, vegetables, and other natural ingredients that owe their vibrant hues to potent antioxidants such as anthocyanins and flavonoids. These compounds not only provide striking colors but also offer a plethora of health benefits, making these foods a valuable addition to any diet.

1. The Power of Anthocyanins:

Anthocyanins are pigments responsible for the blue, purple, and red hues in many fruits and vegetables. Beyond their aesthetic appeal, these compounds boast powerful antioxidant properties that help combat oxidative stress and inflammation in the body. By scavenging harmful free radicals, anthocyanins contribute to cellular health and may reduce the risk of chronic diseases such as heart disease, diabetes, and certain cancers.

2. Exploring Blue and Purple Food:

A. Berries:

Nutritional Benefits:

Blue and purple berries, such as blueberries, blackberries, and elderberries, offer numerous nutritional benefits:

✓ High in Antioxidants:

Blue and purple berries are rich in antioxidants like anthocyanins, which help combat oxidative stress and inflammation in the body, potentially reducing the risk of chronic diseases.

✓ Vitamins and Minerals:

These berries are packed with essential vitamins and minerals, including vitamin C, vitamin K, manganese, and fiber, which support overall health and immune function.

✓ Heart Health:

The compounds found in blue and purple berries may promote heart health by improving cholesterol levels, lowering blood pressure, and reducing the risk of cardiovascular disease.

✓ Brain Health:

Some research suggests that the antioxidants and other compounds in these berries may help improve brain function, protect against age-related cognitive decline, and enhance memory.

✓ Digestive Health:

The fiber content in blue and purple berries supports digestive health by promoting regular bowel movements, preventing constipation, and fostering a healthy gut microbiome.

Incorporating blue and purple berries into your diet can contribute to overall health and well-being due to their nutrient-rich profile and potential health benefits.

B. Purple Vegetables:

Nutritional Benefits:

✓ Antioxidants:

Purple vegetables like purple cabbage, eggplant, and purple potatoes contain anthocyanins, which are powerful antioxidants that help protect cells from damage and reduce inflammation.

✓ Heart Health:

The anthocyanins found in purple vegetables may also help lower the risk of heart disease by improving blood flow, reducing cholesterol levels, and maintaining healthy blood pressure.

✓ Cancer Prevention:

Compounds in purple vegetables, such as flavonoids and phenolic acids, may help reduce the risk of certain types of cancer, including colon and breast cancer.

✓ Eye Health:

Purple vegetables like purple carrots and purple sweet potatoes contain lutein and zeaxanthin, which are important nutrients for eye health.

✓ Brain Function:

The antioxidants in purple vegetables have been linked to improved cognitive function and may help protect the brain from age-related decline. They may also reduce the risk of neurodegenerative diseases like Alzheimer's.

C. Grapes:

Nutritional Benefits:

✓ Resveratrol:

Grapes, especially red and purple varieties, are rich in resveratrol, a powerful antioxidant that has been linked to numerous health benefits, including reducing inflammation and lowering the risk of heart disease.

✓ Heart Health:

The antioxidants and polyphenols in grapes help promote heart health by improving circulation, reducing cholesterol levels, and preventing the oxidation of LDL cholesterol, which can lead to plaque buildup in the arteries.

✓ **Blood Sugar Control**:

Resveratrol and other compounds found in grapes may help improve insulin sensitivity and regulate blood sugar levels, making them beneficial for individuals with diabetes or those at risk of developing the condition.

✓ **Digestive Health**:

Grapes are a good source of fiber, which supports digestive health by promoting regular bowel movements and preventing constipation. Additionally, the polyphenols in grapes may help protect the lining of the digestive tract and reduce the risk of digestive disorders.

✓ **Skin Health:**

The antioxidants in grapes, particularly vitamin C and resveratrol, help protect the skin from damage caused by UV radiation, pollution, and oxidative stress. They may also help reduce the signs of aging, such as wrinkles and fine lines, and promote a healthy, glowing complexion.

D. Purple Grains:

Nutritional Benefits:

Purple grains, such as purple rice, purple barley, and purple corn, offer several nutritional benefits:

✓ **Antioxidants**:
Purple grains are rich in anthocyanins, the pigments responsible for their vibrant color.

Anthocyanins are powerful antioxidants that help protect cells from damage caused by free radicals, reducing the risk of chronic diseases like heart disease and cancer.

✓ **Fiber:**

Like their counterparts, purple grains are high in dietary fiber, which aids digestion, promotes gut health, and helps regulate blood sugar levels. Consuming foods rich in fiber can also contribute to weight management and reduce the risk of obesity.

✓ **Vitamins and Minerals:**

Purple grains contain essential vitamins and minerals, including vitamin E, vitamin B6, potassium, and magnesium. These nutrients are important for overall health, supporting functions such as immune system function, nerve function, and bone health.

✓ Heart Health:

The antioxidants and fiber found in purple grains can help lower cholesterol levels and improve heart health. Regular consumption of these grains may reduce the risk of cardiovascular diseases, such as heart attacks and strokes.

✓ Anti-inflammatory Properties:

Compounds present in purple grains may have anti-inflammatory effects, which can help reduce inflammation in the body and alleviate symptoms of inflammatory conditions like arthritis and inflammatory bowel disease.

3. **Incorporating Blue and Purple Foods into Your Diet**:

Now that we understand the numerous health benefits of blue and purple foods, let's explore some delicious ways to incorporate them into your daily meals:

A. Berries:

Blueberries, blackberries, and raspberries are nutritional powerhouses packed with antioxidants. Enjoy them fresh as a snack, blend them into smoothies, or top your oatmeal or yogurt with a handful of these colorful gems.

B. Purple Vegetables:

Eggplant, purple cabbage, and purple sweet potatoes are excellent sources of vitamins, minerals, and antioxidants. Roast them, sauté them, or add them to salads for a vibrant burst of flavor and nutrition.

C. Grapes:

Whether red or purple, grapes are rich in resveratrol, a potent antioxidant with anti-aging properties. Snack on them whole, freeze them for a refreshing treat, or add them to fruit salads and cheese platters.

D. Purple Grains:

Incorporate nutritious grains like black rice, purple barley, or purple corn into your meals for added fiber and antioxidants. Use them in salads, pilafs, or as a colorful side dish.

Incorporating blue and purple foods into your diet is not only a feast for the senses but also a boon for your health. From protecting your heart and brain to reducing inflammation and fighting cancer, the vibrant pigments and powerful antioxidants found in these foods offer a myriad of health benefits. So, indulge in the rich spectrum of blue and purple foods and embark on a journey towards vibrant health and well-being!

Chapter 6
Violet Harmony - Balancing Your Plate with the Healing Tones of Violet Foods

Welcome to the vibrant world of violet foods, where nature's bounty offers a spectrum of hues that can elevate both your palate and your health. In this chapter, we delve into the significance of violet foods and how incorporating them into your diet can contribute to a balanced and nourished life. Let's embark on a journey of exploration and discovery as we unlock the secrets of violet harmony.

1. Understanding Violet Foods:

Violet foods derive their rich color from natural pigments called anthocyanins, which are potent antioxidants with numerous health benefits. These compounds have been linked to reduced inflammation, improved cardiovascular health, and even potential anti-cancer properties. By incorporating violet foods into your diet, you not only add visual appeal to your meals but also enhance their nutritional value.

2. Exploring of Violet Foods:

A. Purple potatoes:

These vibrant tubers are packed with antioxidants and offer a unique flavor and texture to dishes.

B. Eggplant:

Versatile and delicious, eggplants are a staple in many cuisines, providing fiber, vitamins, and minerals.

C. Blackberries:

Bursting with flavor and nutrients, blackberries are a delicious addition to desserts, smoothies, or enjoyed on their own.

D. Purple cabbage:

With its crisp texture and slightly sweet flavor, purple cabbage is a nutritious addition to salads, stir-fries, or slaws.

E. Plums:

Juicy and sweet, plums are not only delicious but also offer a range of vitamins, minerals, and antioxidants.

3. The Healing Power of Violet Foods:

Violet foods are not just visually stunning; they also possess healing properties that can benefit your body and mind. From supporting heart health to promoting brain function, the nutrients found in violet foods play a crucial role in overall well-being. Let's explore some of the key health benefits associated with incorporating violet foods into your diet:

✓ **Cardiovascular health:**
Anthocyanins found in violet foods have been shown to support heart health by reducing inflammation and improving blood vessel function.

✓ **Brain function:**

Research suggests that the antioxidants in violet foods may help protect brain cells from damage and support cognitive function as we age.

✓ **Cancer prevention**:

Compounds found in violet foods may have anti-cancer properties, although more research is needed in this area.

✓ **Digestive health:**

The fiber content in many violet foods, such as purple cabbage and blackberries, supports digestive health by promoting regularity and gut microbiota balance.

4. Incorporating Violet Foods into Your Diet:

Now that we understand the benefits of violet foods, let's explore some practical ways to incorporate them into your daily meals:

1. Start your day with a vibrant smoothie made with mixed berries, spinach, and a splash of almond milk.
2. Add roasted purple potatoes to salads or serve them as a colorful side dish.
3. Experiment with eggplant in stir-fries, curries, or grilled as a meat substitute.
4. Enjoy a refreshing salad with shredded purple cabbage, carrots, and a tangy vinaigrette.
5. Indulge in the sweetness of fresh plums as a healthy snack or dessert option.

As we conclude our exploration of violet harmony, remember that incorporating a variety of colorful foods into your diet is key to achieving vibrant health and vitality. By embracing the healing tones of violet foods, you not only nourish your body but also indulge your senses in a symphony of flavors and nutrients. Here's to a colorful and nourished life filled with vitality and well-being!

Chapter 7
Beyond the Rainbow - Integrating Colorful Variety for Holistic Wellness

In this chapter, we delve into the profound connection between vibrant colors in our diet and holistic wellness. Just as the colors of the rainbow represent a spectrum of light, incorporating a diverse array of colorful foods into our diet can provide a spectrum of nutrients crucial for optimal health and vitality.

1. Understanding the Rainbow Diet:

The Rainbow Diet is a dietary approach focused on consuming a wide variety of colorful fruits, vegetables, and other plant-based foods. Each color group corresponds to specific phytonutrients, vitamins, and minerals, offering unique health benefits. By embracing the Rainbow Diet, individuals can nourish their bodies with a rich tapestry of nutrients essential for overall well-being.

A. Red Foods:

Foods such as tomatoes, strawberries, and red bell peppers are rich in lycopene, a powerful antioxidant known for its potential to reduce the risk of chronic diseases such as heart disease and certain cancers. Additionally, red foods often contain vitamin C, which supports immune function and collagen production for healthy skin.

B. Orange and Yellow Foods:

Orange and yellow foods like carrots, oranges, and sweet potatoes are abundant in beta-carotene, a precursor to vitamin A that promotes eye health and boosts immune function. These foods also contain vitamin C and flavonoids, which possess anti-inflammatory properties and may support cardiovascular health.

C. **Green Foods**:

Leafy greens such as spinach, kale, and broccoli are packed with chlorophyll, vitamins, and minerals crucial for detoxification and cellular repair. Additionally, green foods provide an abundance of folate, a B vitamin essential for brain health and fetal development during pregnancy.

D. **Blue and Purple Foods:**

Blueberries, purple cabbage, and eggplant are examples of foods rich in anthocyanins, potent antioxidants that help combat oxidative stress and inflammation. Consuming blue and purple foods may support cognitive function, heart health, and overall longevity.

E. Violet foods:

Violet food, also known as purple foods, encompasses a variety of fruits, vegetables, and grains with deep purple or blue-purple hues. Consuming violet foods, such as blueberries, purple cabbage, or eggplant, can contribute to a diverse and nutrient-rich diet, providing essential vitamins, minerals, and phytonutrients that support overall health and well-being. Including a range of colorful foods, including violet ones, is often recommended to maximize nutritional intake and promote a balanced diet.

F. White and Tan Foods:

While often overlooked, white and tan foods like garlic, onions, and cauliflower offer unique health benefits. These foods contain allicin, a sulfur compound with antimicrobial properties, as well as quercetin, a flavonoid that may help reduce inflammation and support immune function.

2. Practical Tips for Embracing the Rainbow Diet:

✓ Aim to include at least one serving of each color group in your meals and snacks throughout the day.

✓ Experiment with new recipes and cooking methods to incorporate a diverse range of colorful ingredients into your diet.

✓ Shop for seasonal produce to ensure freshness and maximize nutritional content.

✓ Consider incorporating smoothies, salads, and bowls as convenient ways to pack multiple colors into one meal.

✓ Embrace mindful eating practices to savor the flavors and textures of your colorful meals, promoting a deeper connection to your food and its nourishing benefits.

By embracing the principles of the Rainbow Diet and incorporating a vibrant spectrum of colors into our meals, we can nourish our bodies, support optimal health, and embark on a journey to a colorful and nourished life. Let the rainbow guide you towards holistic wellness and vitality.

Chapter 8
Recipes Section - Delicious and Nutrient-Packed Rainbow Diet Recipes

Welcome to the Recipes Section of "Unlocking Vibrant Health: The Rainbow Diet Journey to a Colorful and Nourished Life!"This chapter will look at a variety of delicious, nutrient-dense foods that are based on the principles of the Rainbow Diet.Each recipe is carefully crafted to incorporate a vibrant spectrum of colorful fruits, vegetables, and other wholesome ingredients, providing you with a diverse array of nutrients essential for optimal health and well-being.

1. Why the Rainbow Diet?

The Rainbow Diet emphasizes the importance of consuming a wide range of colorful fruits and vegetables to ensure a diverse intake of essential vitamins, minerals, antioxidants, and phytonutrients. By incorporating foods of different colors into your diet, you can maximize the nutritional benefits and support various aspects of your health, including immune function, heart health, digestion, and more.

2. Key Principles of Rainbow Diet Recipes:

A. Color Variety:

Each recipe includes a selection of colorful fruits, vegetables, and other ingredients to provide a diverse range of nutrients.

B. Nutrient Density:

Ingredients chosen for these recipes are nutrient-dense, meaning they offer a high concentration of vitamins, minerals, and other beneficial compounds per calorie.

C. Balance and Moderation:

While the emphasis is on whole, plant-based foods, these recipes also incorporate other essential food groups, such as lean proteins, healthy fats, and whole grains, to ensure a balanced diet.

D. Flavor and Enjoyment:

Eating healthily should also be enjoyable! These recipes are designed to be delicious and satisfying, making it easier to adopt and maintain a nutritious eating pattern.

Now, let's explore some of the mouthwatering recipes that will help you unlock vibrant health on your Rainbow Diet journey.

Recipe 1: Rainbow Veggie Stir-Fry

Ingredients:

- 1 tablespoon olive oil

- 1 onion, thinly sliced

- 2 cloves garlic, minced

- 1 red bell pepper, thinly sliced

- 1 yellow bell pepper, thinly sliced

- 1 cup broccoli florets

- 1 cup sliced carrots

- 1 cup snap peas

- 1 cup sliced purple cabbage

- 2 tablespoons low-sodium soy sauce

- 1 tablespoon rice vinegar

- 1 teaspoon sesame oil

- cooked quinoa or brown rice, ready to be served

Instructions:

1. In a big skillet or wok, warm up the olive oil over medium heat. Add the garlic and onion, and simmer for two to three minutes, or until softened.

2. Add the bell peppers, broccoli, carrots, snap peas, and purple cabbage to the skillet. Cook, stirring frequently, for 5-7 minutes until the vegetables are tender-crisp.

3. Mix the rice vinegar, sesame oil, and soy sauce in a small bowl. After adding the sauce, mix the veggies to ensure an even coating.

4. Cook for an additional 2-3 minutes, stirring constantly, until the sauce has thickened slightly.

5. Serve the stir-fry over cooked brown rice or quinoa for a nutritious and colorful meal.

Nutritional Benefits:

- The variety of colorful vegetables in this stir-fry provides a wide range of vitamins, minerals, and antioxidants.

- Bell peppers are rich in vitamin C, while broccoli and carrots are excellent sources of vitamin A and fiber.

- Purple cabbage contains anthocyanins, powerful antioxidants with anti-inflammatory properties.

- Brown rice or quinoa adds complex carbohydrates and fiber to help keep you feeling full and satisfied.

Enjoy this Rainbow Veggie Stir-Fry as a delicious and nutritious addition to your Rainbow Diet meal rotation!

Recipe 2: Rainbow Fruit Salad

Ingredients:

-Strawberries

-Oranges

-Pineapple

-Kiwi

-Blueberries

-Grapes

Instructions:

1. Wash and prepare all the fruits. Slice the strawberries, oranges, pineapple, kiwi, and grapes as desired.

2. Combine all the sliced fruits in a large bowl and gently toss to mix.

3. Serve immediately or chill in the refrigerator until ready to serve.

Nutritional Benefits:

-This colorful fruit salad is packed with vitamins, minerals, and antioxidants.

-Strawberries provide vitamin C and folate.

-Oranges offer vitamin C and potassium.

-Pineapple contains bromelain which aids digestion.

- Kiwi is rich in vitamin K and fiber.

-Blueberries are high in antioxidants.

-Grapes provide resveratrol which supports heart health.

Enjoy this rainbow fruit salad as a delicious and nutritious addition to your Rainbow Diet meal rotation!

Recipe 3: Quinoa Stuffed Bell Peppers

Ingredients:

-Bell peppers (red, yellow, green)

-Cooked quinoa

-Black beans

- Corn

-Diced tomatoes

 -Onions

-Spices

Instructions:

1. Turn the oven on to 375°F, or 190°C. Slice off the bell peppers' tops, then take out the seeds and membranes.

2. Combine cooked quinoa, black beans, corn, chopped tomatoes, onions, and your preferred spices in a big bowl.

3. Fill the hollowed-out bell peppers with the mixture.

4. Place the stuffed bell peppers in a baking dish and cover with foil.

5. Bake for 25-30 minutes, or until the peppers are tender.

6. Serve hot, optionally garnished with fresh herbs or avocado slices

Nutritional Benefits:
-Bell peppers are rich in vitamin C and antioxidants.

-Quinoa offers complete protein and fiber.

-Black beans provide protein and iron.

-Corn adds fiber and vitamins.

-Diced tomatoes contain lycopene which supports skin health.

-Onions offer flavonoids and sulfur compounds with potential anti-inflammatory properties.

Enjoy this Quinoa Stuffed Bell Peppers
as a delicious and nutritious addition to your Rainbow Diet meal rotation!

Recipe 4: Rainbow Veggie Buddha Bowl

Ingredients:
-Cooked brown rice
-Roasted sweet potatoes (orange)

- Steamed broccoli (green)

- Shredded purple cabbage

-Sliced carrots

- Avocado

-Chickpeas

-Tahini dressing

Instructions:

1. Prepare brown rice as directed on the package.

2. Preheat the oven to 400°F (200°C). Toss sweet potato cubes with olive oil, salt, and pepper, then roast for 20-25 minutes until tender.

3. Steam broccoli until bright green and tender.

4. Assemble bowls with cooked brown rice, roasted sweet potatoes, steamed broccoli,

shredded purple cabbage, sliced carrots, avocado slices, and cooked chickpeas.

5. Drizzle with tahini dressing or your favorite dressing.

6. Serve immediately and enjoy!

Nutritional Benefits:
This Buddha Bowl is a nutrient powerhouse.

-Sweet potatoes are rich in beta-carotene.

- Broccoli provides vitamin K and folate.

-Purple cabbage contains anthocyanins and vitamin C.

-Carrots offer beta-carotene and fiber.

- Avocado provides healthy fats and potassium.

-Chickpeas are high in protein and fiber, and tahini dressing adds calcium and healthy fats.

Enjoy this Rainbow Veggie Buddha Bowl as a delicious and nutritious addition to your Rainbow Diet meal rotation!

Recipe 5: Rainbow Quinoa Salad

Ingredients:

-Cooked rainbow quinoa

- Diced bell peppers (red, yellow, green)

-Cherry tomatoes

Cucumber

-Red onion

-Parsley

-Lemon vinaigrette

Instructions:

1.Cook rainbow quinoa according to package instructions and allow it to cool slightly.

2. In a large bowl, combine cooked quinoa, diced bell peppers, cherry tomatoes, cucumber, red onion, and chopped parsley.

3. Toss the salad with lemon vinaigrette until well combined.

4. Serve immediately, or refrigerate for a few hours to allow flavors to meld before serving.

Nutritional Benefits:

-Quinoa is a complete protein and excellent source of fiber.

-Bell peppers offer vitamin C and antioxidants.

-Cherry tomatoes provide lycopene and vitamin A.

-Cucumber adds hydration and vitamins.

-Red onion offers flavonoids and sulfur compounds.

- Parsley contains vitamin K and antioxidants, and lemon vinaigrette adds flavor and vitamin C.

Enjoy this **Rainbow Quinoa Salad** as a delicious and nutritious addition to your Rainbow Diet meal rotation!

Recipe 6: Rainbow Smoothie Bowl

Ingredients:

-Frozen mixed berries (strawberries, blueberries, raspberries)

-Banana

-Spinach

- Greek yogurt

-Almond milk

- Granola

-Sliced almonds

-Shredded coconut.

Instructions:

1. In a blender, combine frozen mixed berries, bananas, spinach, Greek yogurt, and almond milk.

2. Blend until smooth and creamy, adding more almond milk if needed to reach your desired consistency.

3. Transfer the blended drink to a bowl.

4. Top with granola, sliced almonds, and shredded coconut.

5. Enjoy with a spoon!

Nutritional Benefits:

-This vibrant smoothie bowl is rich in antioxidants, vitamins, and minerals.

- Berries offer vitamin C and fiber.

-Banana adds potassium and natural sweetness.

- Spinach provides iron and vitamin K.

-Greek yogurt offers protein and probiotics.

-Almond milk adds calcium.

-Granola provides whole grains and fiber.

-Sliced almonds offer healthy fats.

- Shredded coconut adds flavor and healthy fats.

Enjoy this **Rainbow Smoothie Bowl** as a delicious and nutritious addition to your Rainbow Diet meal rotation!

These step-by-step instructions will guide you through preparing each Rainbow Diet recipe, allowing you to enjoy delicious and nourishing meals that support your health and well-being.Enjoy experimenting with these colorful and nourishing dishes!

Conclusion

In conclusion, "Unlocking Vibrant Health: The Rainbow Diet Journey to a Colorful and Nourished Life" offers a compelling perspective on achieving long-term health through embracing a colorful lifestyle. Throughout this ebook, we have explored the profound impact of incorporating a diverse range of colorful fruits, vegetables, and whole foods into our diets. By adopting the principles of the Rainbow Diet, readers have been empowered to take charge of their health and embark on a journey toward vitality and well-being.

We have delved into the science behind the Rainbow Diet, uncovering the wealth of nutrients, antioxidants, and phytochemicals present in foods of various hues. From the antioxidant-rich blues and purples of berries to the vitamin-packed oranges and yellows of citrus fruits and carrots, each color spectrum offers unique health benefits that contribute to overall wellness. By incorporating a rainbow of foods into our meals, we can nourish our bodies from the inside out, supporting everything from heart health to immune function.

Furthermore, "Unlocking Vibrant Health" has emphasized the importance of balance and moderation in our dietary choices. While embracing colorful foods forms the foundation of the Rainbow Diet, it is equally essential to prioritize whole, unprocessed foods and to practice mindful eating habits. By listening to our bodies' cues and honoring our nutritional needs, we can cultivate a sustainable approach to healthy living that extends far beyond short-term fads or restrictive diets.Ultimately, the journey towards vibrant health is not just about the foods we eat, but also about the lifestyle choices we make each day. From staying active and prioritizing sleep to managing stress and fostering positive relationships, every aspect of our lives plays a role in shaping our overall well-being. By embracing a holistic approach to health and wellness, readers of "Unlocking Vibrant Health" are empowered to cultivate a life that is not only colorful and nourished but also vibrant and fulfilling.

In closing, I invite readers to embark on their own Rainbow Diet journey, armed with the knowledge and inspiration found within these pages. Together, let us unlock the secrets to vibrant health and embrace a life filled with vitality, joy, and abundance.

Acknowledgments
Gratitude for the Journey of Vibrant Health

Embarking on the journey towards vibrant health through the Rainbow Diet has been a transformative experience filled with gratitude. Gratitude permeates every aspect of this journey, from the colorful array of fruits and vegetables that nourish our bodies to the newfound energy and vitality that accompany improved health.One cannot embark on the Rainbow Diet journey without first acknowledging and embracing gratitude for the opportunity to prioritize health and well-being. Gratitude serves as the foundation upon which this journey is built, grounding us in appreciation for the abundance of nutritious foods available to us and the opportunity to make positive changes in our lives.

Throughout this journey, gratitude acts as a guiding force, reminding us to approach each day with mindfulness and appreciation for the nourishment we provide our bodies. Whether it's savoring the taste and texture of a juicy red apple or reveling in the vibrant hues of a salad filled with leafy greens, gratitude enhances our connection to the food we eat and the impact it has on our health.Moreover, gratitude extends beyond the plate, infusing every aspect of our lives with positivity and appreciation. As we prioritize our health and well-being, we cultivate a deeper sense of gratitude for our bodies and all they allow us to experience. We become more attuned to the signals our bodies send us, more mindful of our habits and behaviors, and more appreciative of the simple joys that life has to offer.

In essence, gratitude is the key that unlocks the door to vibrant health through the Rainbow Diet journey. It reminds us to approach each day with intention and appreciation, to savor the journey, and to celebrate the progress we make along the way. So let us embrace gratitude wholeheartedly as we continue on this colorful and nourishing path towards vibrant health and a more vibrant life.